Treasures Toward Wholeness

Treasures Toward Wholeness

Seeking the Father
for Treasures
and Tools
to become whole -
Physically,
Emotionally,
and Spiritually.

~Rebecca Hazelton

Treasures Toward Wholeness
Rebecca Hazelton

forhisname2@yahoo.com
ISBN: 978-1-941173-34-3

Published by : Olive Press Messianic and Christian Publisher
olivepresspublisher.com

Unless otherwise noted, all scripture references are from the Messianic Jewish Family Bible, Tree of Life Version. Copyright (c) 2015 by the Messianic Jewish Family Bible Society. Used by permission of the Messianic Jewish Family Bible Society." All emphasis is the author's.

CJB – *Complete Jewish Bible* by David H. Stern, copyright © 1998. All rights reserved. Used by permission from Messianic Jewish Publishers, 6120 Day Long Lane, Clarksville, MD 21029.www.messianicjewish.net. All emphasis is the author's.

* Glossary:

Adonai – Hebrew word for Lord, used in place of YHVH in most English translations of the Bible.

Elohim – Hebrew word for God.

Mitzvot – Hebrew word for Commandments

Ruach Hakodesh– Hebrew words for Holy Spirit.

Torah – Hebrew word that means instructions or teaching – often (mis)translated as "law".

Yeshua – Hebrew given name of the Savior redeemer known in English as Jesus. (Yeshua is a shortened form of Yehoshua)

YHVH – Acronym of the Hebrew letters Yud, Hey, Vav, Hey (יהוה (- The 4 letter Tetragramation of the personal name of Elohim (God) from Exodus 3:15. *(I am not indicating any pronunciation of this name. I simply want to acknowledge that my Heavenly Father has a personal name.)*

You search and you know me.
You know my lying down, and my rising up.
You understand my thoughts from afar
and You're acquainted with all my ways.

In the secret place of my mother's womb,
You saw me and everything You knew.
There you took Your time to
    patiently mold me
Every thought is divine.

So I praise You, yes I do.
I am fearfully and wonderfully
    made to be like You.
I praise You, yes I do.
How marvelous and wonderful
    is everything You do.

It was so ordinary the way I came to be,
Boy to man and now, here I stand.
Now I've come to realize,
There's much more to me,
I'm a son of Elohim*.

And I praise You, yes I do.
I am fearfully and wonderfully
    made to be like You.
I praise You, yes I do,

Here's just one tiny grain of sand
   in an ocean of Your thoughts for me.

Where can I go from your spirit?
Where can I flee from you?
For when I'm awake I find I'm still with You.

I praise You, yes I do
How marvelous and wonderful
   is everything You do.
I praise You, yes I do
From before there was time,
Every day you had in mind.
I praise You, yes I do
Here's just one tiny grain of sand
   in an ocean of Your thoughts for me.

I came from You , So I go back to You
Cuz where You are is where I want to be.

I praise You….. I praise You……..Praise You

(Psalm 139 – "Selah Vol. 1" James Block © 2014
www.selahmusic.org also found on Youtube.com)

Contents

~ Introduction ~

"Yes, if you call out for insight, lifting up your voice for discernment, if you seek her as silver and search for her as for <u>hidden treasures,</u> then you will know the fear of Adonai and discover the knowledge of God. For Adonai gives wisdom. Out of His mouth comes knowledge and understanding."(Proverbs 2:3-6)

"I pray that from the <u>treasures</u> of His glory, He will empower you with inner strength by His Spirit, so that the Messiah may live in your hearts through your trusting." (Ephesians 3:16,17 CJB)

Years ago I began to "inquire of the Lord" about things pertaining to my health. In my quest I have been given some "treasures" from YHVH* that have helped me along my path to understanding. Being without the world's insurance definitely has given me more impetus to search deeper when I encounter a physical problem. However, in sharing these treasures with you, I want to clarify that this is a very personal journey.

Each of us have challenges in our lives. Physically, emotionally or spiritually. Some of these challenges are self-created by choices we have made and sin(s) we have committed or are living in. (See an example in Psalms 38 and 51) Some are products of the "fallen" world we live in and what mankind is destructively doing to itself. Some are a result of heritage and/or what others have done to us. We also have an adversary, an enemy of Elohim* and our souls. We or our forefathers may have "opened a door" to his involvement in our lives, knowingly or unknowingly. Finally, you may have been born with a physical challenge that has nothing to do with any of the above. See John 9:1-4

I do not believe it is YHVH's desire that we are or become sick. I believe He desires for us to be well and has set up a way for us to be well. He might send plagues and pestilence as judgment on peoples and nations when we disobey His commands. We cannot deny that we may experience trials under judgment as He attempts to return us to holiness. We even see an example in the book of Job when YHVH allows the adversary to test Job. Regardless of the reason, He wants to use each challenge, no matter what kind it is or what source it is from, to draw us into a deeper relationship with Him - to teach us of His ways, to mature us, and bring us into His fullness. We make choices each day how we will apply what He teaches us and how we will live out His particular calling and purposes for our lives.

In that very individual relationship that He desires to have with us, we should be inquiring of Him first when it comes to our health. There is no one who knows everything about us (including doctors). No person knows our bodies, our hearts, our thoughts, our past, or our future. Only YHVH. As it states in Psalm 139 *"You are intimately acquainted with all my ways."* (vs 3 - CJB) This wonderful Psalm about the intimacy our Creator desires to have with us ends with these words. *"Examine me, God and know my heart. Test me, and know my thoughts. See if there is in me any hurtful way, and lead me along the eternal ways."* (vs. 23,24 - CJB) What an appropriate way to begin our quest for health and wholeness.

****

There are three parts of our being. Physical, Emotional, and Spiritual. They work in harmony with each other. If one part is sick, the other two will respond. Our bodies usually manifest the sickness and we call it disease. The word itself points to its origin. Dis – ease. What YHVH wants to do is to reveal to us what part of us is not at "ease" or in health and bring us to wholeness and completeness. In other words - a complete Shalom. (The word Shalom in Hebrew, which is often translated as peace, literally means wholeness and completeness.)

There are many resources that shed light on this area of study. Some sources deal with the **Spiritual Roots of Disease**. Another avenue of study is what is happening to the cells in our bodies and the **Physical Roots of Disease.** There are so many resources "out there" that one can get overwhelmed with the possibilities and opinions by all kinds of "experts". I am no expert, by any means, but what I plan to share is my own simple list of treasures or tools that I feel have helped me along a path to wholeness and wellness. This is by no means a complete list or story. It is just a glimpse to hopefully inspire you to do your own search. I will make a few recommendations at the end of this little epistle, but you need to find your own way through the maze of options, hopefully as led by the Spirit of YHVH.

Some may be asking "How do you hear from God? How do I know what I am thinking is from Him?" In the book of John, chapter 10, Yeshua* refers to Himself as "the good shepherd". He says *"the sheep follow [Me] because they know [My] voice. They will never follow a stranger, but will run away from him, for they do not know the voice of strangers."* (John 10:4b,5) Consider when you have a personal friend or family member who calls you on the telephone. They do not need to announce who is calling because we know their voice. We are very familiar with it because we have spent time with them. We know how they speak and what kinds of things they would say. If we are "His sheep", then we want to spend time with the Shepherd, listening to the kinds of things He would say to us from His Word (the Bible). It has been given to us as an instruction book – a *"Torah"** – instructions for life. He has also given us His ***Ruach HaKodesh**** (Holy Spirit) who has been promised to *"teach us all things."* (John 14:26 -KJB) Anything He says will match up to His Word. The more familiar you are with the original the better you will be able to discern a counterfeit.

Another litmus test for whether something is from YHVH or not is what fruit it produces in us. Is it producing the *"peaceful fruit of righteousness"*? (Hebrews 12:11) Is it building character in us? Is it drawing us into more dependence on the Father? Do we have the *"shalom which surpasses all understanding?"* (Philippians 4:7) Or is there confusion, chaos, destruction, strife, despair, hopelessness?

These are important questions to ask ourselves. As you read about the treasures in my own box, I invite you to journal and consider your own journey toward health and wholeness. I believe YHVH wants to give you a specific, very personal "strategy" for your healing. My tools may not be your tools. My journey is not your journey. Again, this is meant to be an inspiration, not an answer. You need to seek YHVH for your own personalized strategy. Seek the face of the Father for His help. (If you don't have a relationship with YHVH, may I invite you to ask Him to reveal Himself to you and begin the most important relationship you will ever have? One that brings life – life everlasting! (John 3:16))

Questions to Consider:

Do I have a personal relationship with YHVH? (Am I "born again"? See John 3)

Do I know my Shepherd's voice?

Do I choose daily whom I will serve?

Do I spend time with and am I willing to ask YHVH to examine me and test me to see what is in my heart?

Is my life displaying the "peaceful fruit of righteousness"? or Is there chaos, destruction, confusion, strife, despair or hopelessness in my life or family?

Have I sought YHVH for **His** strategy for my health/life?

What have I learned from this Introduction?

~Treasure #1~
"Why do you want to be sick?"

"Now a certain man had been an invalid there for thirty-eight years. Seeing him lying there and knowing he had been that way a long time, Yeshua said to him, <u>"Do you want to get well?"</u> (John 5:5-6)

And here two blind men sitting by the roadside, when they heard that Yeshua was passing by, cried out, saying, "Have mercy on us, O Master, Ben-David!" The crowd warned them to be quiet, but they cried out all the more, saying, "Have mercy on us, O Master, Ben-David!" Yeshua stopped and called out to them. <u>"What do you want Me to do for you?"</u> He said. They said to Him, "Master, let our eyes be opened!" Moved with compassion, Yeshua touched their eyes. Instantly they regained their sight and followed Him." (Matthew 20:30-34)

About twenty years ago I was going through an unexpected, undesired divorce, trying to find ways to provide for my two teenage daughters. I was working, sometimes in excess of 50 hours a week. I was angry and hurt by my husband's desertion. In addition, I was sick. I didn't have time to be sick. I didn't have the energy to even think about being sick. But I could not deny that what I was experiencing was beyond my control. In my desperation I was going to a counselor who also happened to be a very good friend. He asked me a very poignant question. *"Why do you want to be sick?"* Of course I rebutted *"I don't want to be sick. I don't have time to be sick. Why would you even ask that question?"* He just smiled and asked if I would consider it.

That question haunted me for the year in which I sought answers to my evasive symptoms which acted very much like chronic fatigue syndrome. (It turned out that I had mercury poisoning from very old and deep fillings in my teeth which was seeping into my blood stream and affecting every area of my body.)

One time while I was driving home from an appointment with my naturopathic doctor, the truth hit me. *"I want someone to take care of me. I want to be sick so someone will take care of me!"* I knew then that I had somehow allowed this sickness. My subconscious plan was not working. The longer it went on the more frustrated I became. Each step forward ended up in two steps behind. As I uncovered this truth, I began to come to grips with reality, beginning the tedious journey of facing my own "demons" and being willing to ask myself the hard questions.

No wonder my body was sick! I was emotionally devastated and spiritually not right with my creator. I was angry at God. He was the one that told me to marry this man! I began to realize that my dis-ease was deeper than the physical symptoms and the causes I was experiencing. I needed to get right with God first, then forgive myself for going astray, forgive my ex-husband, and do what I needed to do physically to help my body heal. I had my mouth redone and the mercury and other heavy metals removed from my system, but I also began to remove some spiritual and emotional poison as well. It was shortly after that that I began to heal. It was a combination of learning, not only the root cause of my sickness physically, but the root cause emotionally, and spiritually too. I also decided that I needed to be well for the sake of my daughters and sought for it with a passion.

"Surely You desire truth in the inner being. Make me know wisdom inwardly." (Psalm 51;8(6)) "For this reason many among you are weak and sick, and quite a few have died. For if we were judging ourselves thoroughly, we wouldn't be coming under judgment. But when we are judged, we are being disciplined by

the Lord so that we might not be condemned along with the world."(1 Corinthians 11:30-32)

Questions to consider:

What do I think is the major cause of my dis-ease?

Have I asked YHVH to reveal the source of my dis-ease?

Do I want to be well?

What have I asked Yeshua to do for me?

Is there anyone I need to forgive (including myself)?

What have I learned from this treasure?

~ Treasure #2 ~

"The number of days that were ordained for you are set. You can either choose to live them sick or well."

"Your eyes could see me as an embryo, but in Your book all my days were already written; my days had been shaped before any of them existed." (Psalm 139:16 - CJB)

"One's spirit sustains him through illness, but who can bear a crushed spirit?" (Proverbs 18:14)

I had a good friend in High School. She was quiet and like the rest of our "gang" we were the misfits and the "goody two shoes" of our class. As "nerds" we often simply stuck together. No dates. No invitations to the prom. We decided to spend the day of the prom together, ending it with a fancy dinner at a restaurant where we dressed in long gowns and had the time of our lives. We decided that we had had a better time than all the rest of the girls who went with a guy because we didn't have to impress anyone!

It was only a few years ago that I was informed, to my great sadness, that my friend had taken her own life. At the time, I was going through another very difficult season of my own. Something about that news sent me spiraling downward. I was already struggling with thoughts of not wanting to live, but to know that she had not made it scared me. I was in a spiritual battle. The enemy of my soul was enticing me to do the same. *"You feel trapped. Why don't you take the easy way out?"* Was that a thought in my head? I couldn't believe I was listening to his lies, but I also could not get above my feelings of despair.

I was in that state of depression when I received, what I call a "text message" from above. YHVH often "texts" me when He wants my attention. The reason I call it a "text message" is because it seems to run like a ticker tape across my mind. This one said *"The number of days that were ordained for you are set. You can either choose to live them sick or well."* Wow. I was asked to choose sickness or wellness. That was a turning point in my depression. I sought prayer to end the spiritual battle I was in. The depression lifted. I was able to face my difficult time with a new energy to find ways to be well – spiritually, emotionally, and physically.

Have you ever wondered why some people live a long life even though they are very ill? Why do people linger on and on in states of mental, physical, and spiritual disease? Perhaps this is a clue. I don't know how it all works with the Father. I do know that it isn't up to me what is going on in another person's life. I am reminded of a scene after Yeshua has risen from the dead and is back with his disciples. He has just fed them some fish on the shores of the Galilee. He has asked Peter some pretty deep questions about loving and serving when Yeshua begins to tell him what will happen to him at the end of his life. *"Yes, indeed! I tell you, when you grow old, you will stretch out your hands, and someone else will dress you and carry you where you do not want to go."* (John 21:18) Shortly after that Peter asks Yeshua *"Lord, what about him?"* (vs 21) referring to John. Yeshua's reply is right to the point. *"If I want him to stay on until I come, what is it to you? You, follow Me!"* (vs 22) It must have felt like a slap on the face, but sometimes we need to hear that same word. It is a command that all that matters is that we follow Him. What happens with others is really none of our business.

Questions to consider:

What do I believe about depression? Is it a Biblical concept?

Do I spend time worrying about my health?

Do I spend time comparing myself to other people?

Am I a follower of Yeshua or a follower of man?

Do I judge other people and concern myself with their situations?

What have I learned from this treasure?

~ Treasure #3 ~

" "So she [Rivka] went to inquire of Adonai" (Genesis 25:22)

"The Spirit of Adonai Elohim is on me, because Adonai has anointed me to proclaim Good News to the poor. He has sent me to bind up the brokenhearted, to proclaim liberty to the captives, and the opening of the prison to those who are bound, to proclaim the year of Adonai's favor and the day of our God's vengeance, to comfort all who mourn to console those who mourn in Zion, to give them beauty for ashes, the oil of joy for mourning, the garment of praise for the spirit of heaviness, that they might be called oaks of righteousness, the planting of Adonai, that He may be glorified." (Isaiah 61:1-3 and Luke 4:18,19)

When Rivka (Rebekah) was troubled about what was going on in her body, the Bible indicates that she inquired of Adonai first. It doesn't say she went to her doctor or asked her neighbor or even her midwife. She asked the creator of the universe what was going on with her body (and the warring unborn within her.)

I was experiencing shortness of breath and coughing. My symptoms were very much like asthma. It was getting worse. We found out that there was mold in the apartment we were living in, which I was allergic to. Even though the physical situation was remedied, my asthma did not improve. Even after leaving the apartment for a time, I did not have relief. My family wanted me to go to a doctor. I had to be firm, but said *"I won't go until I get word from my heavenly Father."* I was learning from my "name sake" ancestor Rivka that I needed to "inquire of Adonai" first before seeking other avenues of healing.

19

I went into prayer and fasting to seek the Lord. After a few days He showed me why I couldn't breathe. It was the result of something someone had done to hurt me several years before. Even though I had never had physical symptoms as a result of the incident, the spiritual and emotional scars were there that "opened a door" for the struggle to breathe. As soon as I recognized the root of my dis-ease, I forgave again, the person that injured me. I prayed for God to heal that memory. Immediately I felt the symptoms of asthma lessen and within a week I was breathing normally. I still had a mold allergy, but it did not have a hold on me. *"He that gets wisdom, loves his own soul, He that keeps understanding shall find good."* (Proverbs 19:8)

I believe that most of the time we do not appropriate what is available to us. We have bought into the world's system of health. We do not inquire of YHVH first as Rivka did. We have come to rely so much on the world's system that we have no patience until the Lord reveals the answer to us! Sometimes it takes great perseverance and patience to hear. Sometimes the answers are not what we want to hear! Sometimes the trial is to test what is in our hearts....but!.... I believe there **is** an answer and **only** YHVH knows what it is and how **He** wants to deal with it. YHVH gave us many tools for health. Some of them are shunned by the world because the world's system is all based on prestige, power, and money. YHVH's system is provision through various sources. Some of them are natural. Simple. Easy. Sometimes they are through the medical profession, but we should inquire of YHVH first, not when we have exhausted our human effort.

We must also consider how much we really trust YHVH. When we are not trusting in the creator of the universe who knows everything, we are being our own little "gods" who think we know better. That is idolatry. Or, we don't believe He knows what is best for us. Or a million other excuses. That is why unbelief is sin. (Romans 14:23b *"...whatever is not of faith is sin."*) Sometimes it is rebellion and that is equal to the sin of witchcraft! *"Let us examine ourselves....."*

Questions to consider:

Who do I go to first when I feel sick?

Who do I trust will heal me? Doctors? Medicine? YHVH?

Am I dependent on the health care system to take care of my physical needs? (Or even on natural remedies!)

Do I take time to listen to YHVH to give me instructions and strategy concerning my health?

How much do I really trust YHVH?

What have I learned from this treasure?

~ Treasure #4 ~

"I believe God can change the molecular structure so that it will be nourishing to us."

"For everything created by God is good, and nothing is to be rejected if it is received with thanksgiving; for it is sanctified through the word of God and prayer." (1 Timothy 4:4-5)

I was participating in a prison ministry week in Alabama. As a team, we would enter the women's work release prison in the morning to spend the day with the inmates. We would have lunch with them, even eating the prison food. The first day we sat to dine with them, the inmates wanted to know why on earth we would eat the food in front of us. To them, it was disgusting, but it was all they had. (To be honest, it was not what I would personally order in a restaurant. A lot of starch and not many vitamins.) They felt we had a choice.

I found myself saying. *"Well, there are three reasons. The first reason is because before me is more food than most of the people on the earth have to eat today and I will be thankful for it. Secondly, there is no reason to eat different food from you because we are here to be among you, not to be better than you. And thirdly, I believe God can change the molecular structure of the food so that it will be nourishing to us!"* The first two received nods, but after the third one, one inmate quipped *"You are crazy!"* I admitted that I probably was, but after I said that, I had to think to myself – Do I really believe that? Do I really believe that God can do that?

We live in a broken world that is decaying in front of our eyes. Our food sources have been modified and compromised. Our air is polluted. Our water is so polluted it is treated with many chemicals. We fill our bodies with synthetic drugs that mask symptoms, but never really cure anything, causing side effects which require more drugs. The cycle goes on and on. The cells of our bodies are starved for nutrition. They are screaming at us with aches, pains, and chronic dis-eases. When we look up, we see chemical clouds in strips and blocks which we know is not normal. Surely those chemicals are not staying above, but sinking into our ground and water supplies. There cannot be a truly organic field anymore.

Many people are resorting to "organic" and natural products, but not everyone can afford that expensive transition. What is truly organic? What do we do? *"For everything created by God is good, and nothing is to be rejected if it is received with thanksgiving; for it is sanctified through the word of God and prayer."* (I Timothy 4:4) How are we to interpret this verse? I don't believe it gives us license to eat whatever we want whenever we want to. *"Or don't you know that your body is a temple of the Ruach ha-Kodesh who is in you, whom you have from God, and that you are not your own? (1 Corinthians 6:19) If anyone destroys God's temple, God will destroy him; for God's temple is holy, and you are that temple. (1 Corinthians 3:17)* These verses seem to indicate that we should be careful how we treat our "temple" – referring to our bodies. If we view our bodies as a "temple" of the Ruach HaKodesh – the *Holy* Spirit of Elohim, then should we not be concerned about what we are allowing entrance to that temple as to not "defile" it? Part of our sanctification should be in the area of food consumption. We *should* be very careful what we eat and drink.

I personally believe we have been given some instructions concerning food in the Word of God that we should pay attention to. Many who have returned to a Biblical diet have found restored health to their bodies. Years ago I saw the wisdom of YHVH in restricting pork and certain scavenging shell fish and birds from our diets. YHVH is all about LIFE. Those creatures eat anything – including dead things. The animals that He considers clean ("kosher") are plant eating, not scavengers. (Just a note: Peter's Acts 10 vision is not about food – it is about people).

I also try to stay away from the most offending substances that are known to clog us up like refined (white) flours and sugars, chemical sweeteners, hydrogenated oils, high fructose corn syrup, and preservatives. I read labels and try to cook from scratch. I try not to use processed foods as much as possible. I am trying to do my part in being careful with what I take into my own body and feed my family.

At the same time I am also trusting YHVH to take what I do eat and make it nourishing to my body and to take care of these bodies that are subject to what man has done to what we eat, breathe, and drink. I am truly thankful that I have food to eat, in such an abundant variety. I want to be a good steward of what I am given.

I also believe we have been given a great many promises of health and wellbeing in the Word of God. I believe reciting and personalizing Psalm 91 each day is a way to acknowledge that YHVH is the source of my protection from the attacks of pestilence and plague and every "snare" the enemy would want to use to *"steal, kill, and destroy"* mankind - especially YHVH's chosen ones. As I uncover each treasure, I realize that I can live my life to its fullest measure. *"The thief comes only to steal, slaughter, and destroy. I have come that they might have life, and have it abundantly!"* (John 10:10)

Questions to consider:

Am I truly grateful for what YHVH has provided for me?

Have I ever considered His list of "clean and unclean" food as pertaining to my "temple"?

Am I careful to read labels and avoid food that is not good for me?

Am I being a good steward of this earth that He has given us to dwell in?

Do I believe YHVH can really change DNA? Both in food and in my body?

What have I learned from this treasure?

~ Treasure #5 ~

"Speak Life into his dying body"

"We know that the tent which houses us here on earth is torn down, we have a permanent building from God, a building not made by human hands, to house us in heaven. For in this tent, our earthly body, we groan with desire to have around us the home from heaven that will be ours. With this around us we will not be found naked. Yes, while we are in this body, we groan with the sense of being oppressed; it is not so much that we want to take something off, but rather to put something on over it; _so that what must die may be swallowed up by the Life_. Moreover, it is God who has prepared us for this very thing, and as a pledge he has given us his Spirit. So we are always confident – we know that so long as we are at home in the body, we are away from our home with the Lord; for we live by trust, not by what we see. We are confident, then, and would much prefer to leave our home in the body and come to our home with the Lord." (2 Corinthians 5: 1-8 – CJB)

"Everybody wants to go to heaven, but nobody wants to die" (Song by Loretta Lynn)

My dad suffered from an arterial disease that blocked the blood flow to his lower extremities. Correcting this situation was not in time for healing to come to some pretty major ulcers that had developed in his feet. Within a short time infection set in. He was facing amputation of both of his lower legs. A very stoic man, my father lived another 5 years, even learning to walk with prosthetics and continue his Uncle Sam performances. Veterans at the VA hospitals welcomed him because he was able to encourage men who had also lost limbs. My dad's motto was *"I'm blessed. I'm blessed. I'm blessed."*

I believe his attitude during these very difficult and suffering years taught me much about being thankful. It was during the last few months of his life, in the winter/spring of 2009, that I was able to be by his side as he was suffering from the same disease. Now his stumps were infected. There was nothing that could be done. He was facing his last days.

It was an honor to sit by his side in the middle of the night. I would serve him a "hot toddy" (hot lemon and honey) and a few crackers when he could not sleep. He would tell me stories of when he was young and foolish. We laughed and cried together. I wondered what I would have missed had I not been willing to get up in the middle of the night to sit with him.

It was also during that time, the Lord showed me how to pray for him. He told me to speak life into his dying body. I wondered why. I saw his eminent death and how much he was suffering. He was not afraid to die, although he cried because he didn't want to leave his bride of almost 65 years. I wanted understanding. The Father told me *"Because he will go from life to life. You speak life into him because death has no sting. Life is what I am about."* In the verse quoted above we see the confirmation of this - *"so that what must die may be swallowed up by the Life."* How precious a thought.

I have learned to speak life into people, myself, and even inanimate objects, like my car. I drove my 1998 Saturn SL2 to 246,000 miles without a major overhaul or breakdown. Every thousand miles we would pause to pray over the car, thanking the Lord for each mile and praying life into each moving part. Some people speak to plants. Did you ever notice that a house that isn't lived in "dies"? It begins to deteriorate and fall apart. Without life, we die.

There are three major things that bring life. Love, blessings, and light. (YHVH and Yeshua embody all three!) There is a powerful verse in Proverbs 18:21 *"Life and death are in the power of the tongue."* And from Psalm 34 - *"Whoever wants to love life and see good days must keep his tongue from evil and his lips from speaking deceit, turn from evil and do good, seek peace and chase after it. For Adonai keeps his eyes on the righteous, and his ears are open to their prayers; but the face of Adonai is against those who do evil things."* (I Peter 3:10-12) We must be so careful what we "confess" - what comes out of our mouths. I am learning to speak life and blessings, inviting the light of Yeshua into everyone I meet and into every situation I encounter. *"Pleasant words are like a honeycomb, sweet to the taste, healing for the body."* (Proverbs 16:24)

Questions to consider:

Am I afraid to die?

Do I believe we go from "life to life" and that death has no sting?

Am I careful what I "confess" with my mouth concerning my health?

Am I thankful for everything?

What have I learned from this treasure?

~ Treasure #6 ~

Commanding my body and soul!

"Of David. Bless Adonai, O my soul, and all that is within me, bless His holy Name. Bless Adonai, O my soul, and forget not all His benefits: He forgives all your iniquity. He heals all your diseases. He redeems your life from the Pit. He crowns you with lovingkindness and compassions. He satisfies your years with good things, so that your youth is renewed like an eagle." (Psalms 103:1-5)

"For although we do live in the world, we do not wage war in a worldly way, because the weapons we use to wage war are not worldly. On the contrary, they have God's power for demolishing strongholds. We demolish arguments and every arrogance [imagination] that raises itself up against the knowledge of God; we take every thought captive and make it obey the Messiah..." (2 Corinthians 10:5,6 - CJB)

..... choose for yourselves today whom you will serve.... But as for me and my household, we will worship Adonai!" (Joshua 24:14-15)

Our journey along this life is a daily choice of whom we will serve. Will I submit myself to YHVH and serve Him? Or - Will I serve myself and my own desires (which fulfills the desire of the adversary)?! (See Genesis 3) There are really only two choices. Only two kingdoms. Light and Dark. Which kingdom am I a citizen of? There are really only two kinds of people. Redeemed and unredeemed. If I am a citizen of the kingdom of Light, then my "spirit" is transformed and I am "redeemed". The rest of me, my mind, will, and emotions are in need of being redeemed or perfected. I like the old word – sanctified. Will I allow the Ruach of YHVH to perfect my soul or will I follow my "carnal" (selfish) nature? (Romans 8)

Now my body is a part of fallen man and will die. There is no choice in that matter, however, I do not need to let my body rule my soul and cloud my spirit! I believe we can command our souls and bodies to "Bless the Lord!" The Hebrew word for "bless" is "baruch". It literally means to "bow the knee"! I have learned to take authority over my soul and body by commanding every cell to *"bow the knee to the Lordship of Yeshua"* and to *"come into alignment with the will of YHVH."* I will not let my emotions, my will or my mind rule me. My spirit man must be the one who decides how the rest of "us" is going to follow through on a given day.

One of the most powerful verses to consider is: *"And if the **Ruach** [Spirit] **of the One who raised Yeshua from the dead dwells in you,** [then] **the One who raised Messiah Yeshua from the dead will also give life to your mortal bodies through His Ruach** [Spirit] **who dwells in you."** (Romans 8:11) This verse confirms that our spirit, which, if in union with the Spirit of YHVH can affect our mortal bodies. A few verses before this one we see how our mind should be set on "things above" and not let our "old nature" rule our minds and spirits.

Every morning I begin my day by thanking and praising YHVH. *"I will enter His gates with Thanksgiving in my heart. I will enter His courts with praise."* (Psalm 100:4) *"But you are holy, you who inhabit the praises of Israel."* (Psalm 22:4(3)). I thank Him for giving me life, for opening my eyes, and for everything I can think of! I recite scriptures and sing out songs that declare who YHVH is. *"Who is like unto You, O Yah, among the gods. Who is like You? Glorious in Holiness. Fearful in praises. Doing wonders. Who is like unto You!"* (From Exodus 15:11) Then I give myself to YHVH, asking Him to order my day according to His will. I surrender my mind, will, and emotions to Him. (Romans 12:1,2) I ask him to "take captive" my thoughts. I "cast down" my imaginations (and I have a vivid imagination!) (II Corinthians 10:3-6). If I have a particular ailment or complaint that my body is shouting at me, I command my cells to bow the knee to the Lordship of Yeshua and come into alignment with the will of YHVH. I recite Psalm 91. I thank Yeshua for His sacrifice and blood shed for me. Then I use the authority He has given me to cancel assignments the enemy might have against me, my marriage, my husband, my family, and those in my personal and spiritual jurisdiction. I claim a "lamb for a household" and cover my children and grandchildren. I bind spiritual powers of darkness and everything that exalts itself against the knowledge of YHVH.

This does not mean that instantaneously I am well and have a great day. It just means that I am purposing myself to be lined up with the Kingdom of Light, not allowing the Kingdom of Darkness to rule over me! I am putting myself in a position of listening to my creator for His instructions for my day. How does He want me to take care of the things that are not yet redeemed in my world? I call those things "unredeemed parts". I want to present myself before Him as a bride without spot or wrinkle. I want my mind to be filled with those things that bring life and blessing. The key is LIFE! It is what YHVH is all about. Life. And even when we pass on, we are passing from Life to Life if we are His. So, if I have passed on from this world's life, know that it was YHVH who allowed my passing, that it was my time, and that I am now in the REAL REAL! Life. Hallelujah!!!! Rejoice.

Rejoice in the Lord always—again I will say, rejoice! Let your gentleness be known to all people. The Lord is near. <u>Do not be anxious [worry] about anything</u>—but in everything, by prayer and petition <u>with thanksgiving</u>, let your requests be made known to God. (Why worry when you can pray!) *And the shalom of God, which surpasses all understanding,* *will guard your hearts and your minds in Messiah Yeshua. Finally, brothers and sisters, whatever is true, whatever is honorable, whatever is just, whatever is pure, whatever is lovely, whatever is commendable—if there is any virtue and if there is anything worthy of praise—dwell on these things.* (Philippians 4:4-8) Amen!

Questions to consider:

Do I believe that YHVH can heal ALL my diseases?

Do I bless my body or speak badly about it?

Does my body rule my spirit or does my spirit rule my body?

How do I begin my day? Do I present myself as a *"living sacrifice"* which is my *"reasonable service"*? (Romans 12:1) Do I want to be *"transformed by the renewing of my mind?"* (Romans 12:2)

Do I ask YHVH to "take captive" my thoughts? Do I allow my imagination to "worry" about my health?

Do I want to be perfected by YHVH and presented before Him without spot or wrinkle?

What have I learned from this treasure?

~ Treasure #7 ~

Light into Soul wounds

"Yeshua spoke to them again, saying, "I am the light of the world. The one who follows Me will no longer walk in darkness, but will have the <u>light of life.</u>" (John 8:12)

For this reason also, ever since we heard about you, we have not stopped praying for you. We keep asking God that you might be filled with the knowledge of His will in all wisdom and spiritual understanding— to walk in a manner worthy of the Lord, to please Him in all respects, bearing fruit in every good work and growing in the knowledge of God. We pray that you may be strengthened with all the power that comes from His glorious might, for you to have all kinds of patience and steadfastness. With joy we give thanks to the Father, who qualified you to share in the inheritance of the kedoshim (holy ones) in the light. <u>He rescued us from the domain of darkness and brought us into the kingdom of the Son whom He loves.</u> (Colossians 1:9-13)

For once you were darkness, but now in union with the Lord you are light. <u>Walk as children of light</u> (for the fruit of light is in all goodness and righteousness and truth), trying to learn what is pleasing to the Lord. Take no part in the fruitless deeds of darkness, but rather expose them— for it is disgraceful even to mention the things that are done by them in secret. Yet everything exposed by the light is being made visible, for everything made visible is light…. So pay close attention to how you walk—not as unwise people but as wise. Make the most of your time because the days are evil. For this reason do not be foolish, but understand what the Lord's will is. (Ephesians 5:8-17)

During our many travels across the USA, as well as Israel, I have picked up certain books or listened to certain teachings which have enhanced what the Father is already in the process of teaching me. I see Him confirm what He is teaching me through what He is teaching others as well. I want to be teachable, so I glean from my brothers and sisters in Messiah truths they have been given, knowing that it is all subject to scrutiny against the Word of YHVH. Several years ago I listened to a teaching series by Katie Souza entitled "The Healing School". In her series of teachings she explains "soul wounds" and their effect on us. She has been given the "treasure" of seeing the Light of Yeshua as the healing source of these soul wounds. This healing brings freedom to those of us who have been bound in some way or another. I began to ask YHVH to shine His light on my soul to expose any darkness that might be lurking there.

One thing that I needed to do in this period of time was to break soul ties I had with past relationships. I allowed the Ruach HaKodesh to expose any unhealthy soul ties I had to men in my past, repenting of anything that I had done to open my heart to anyone who was not meant to be my soul mate for life. I had dreams that helped me see those soul connections. I asked Yeshua to shine His light on those events and relationships, cleansing me from them. It was very freeing. I believe it allowed me to focus my attention and affections on my husband even more. It is a clean feeling, not being attached to anyone else in this world but only that one which the Father ordained for me to be "one" with.

I did a study on Light in the Bible. It is amazing the number of verses that speak of Light. I am fascinated by learning the original Biblical language of Hebrew. There is so much to learn. It is unending. The language is pictorial. In every verse there are layers of meaning. To learn the root of Hebrew words opens up a whole world of understanding the scriptures! (In fact, every translation of the Bible is a paraphrase – many of the true and original meanings have been lost in translation. See my book "For His Name Yeshua")

Light is a key in the first chapter of Genesis. Actually, the literal Hebrew of Genesis 1:3 says *"BE LIGHT!"* vs 4 *"God saw that the light was good, and God divided the light from the darkness."* Did you know that light is "divided" from darkness on Day 1, but the sun and moon, what we consider the source of physical light, were not created until the 4th day? So, the light of Day One must be a spiritual light. Many people believe that the days of creation are connected to the millenniums of the world. The 4th day of creation, if we connect that to the 4th millennium, would correlate to the "Light of the World" coming onto the world's stage. John speaks of this Light in his first chapter and expounds on the Light being the Word and being Life. *"In the beginning was the Word. The Word was with God, and the Word was God. He was with God in the beginning. All things were made through Him, and apart from Him nothing was made that has come into being. In Him was life, and the life was the light of men. The light shines in the darkness, and the darkness has not overpowered it…. The true light, coming into the world, gives light to every man."* (John 1:1-5,9) Yeshua is the Light of the World!

Questions to consider:

Am I teachable?

Am I careful what I read? Do I allow YHVH to guide my choice of books, teaching, and other media options?

Do I read the Bible more than other books?

What soul wounds do I have?

What unhealthy soul connections do I need to repent of and break?

Am I aware of the origins of the Bible and its Hebrew language and culture?

What have I learned from this treasure?

~ Treasure #8 ~

"What legal right does the enemy have to torment me?"

"......because the ruler of this world is coming. He has no claim on me." (CJB) ("For the prince of this world cometh, and hath nothing in me." KJV) (John 14:30)

"Don't bring something abhorrent into your house, or you will share in the curse that is on it; instead, you are to detest it completely, loathe it utterly; for it is set apart for destruction." (Deuteronomy 7:26 - CJB)

"And there was a woman with a blood flow for twelve years, who could not be healed by anyone. She came up from behind and touched the tzitzit (wings) of Yeshua's garment. Immediately, her blood flow stopped." (Luke 8:43-44)

Several years ago the John 14 verse "popped out" as I was reading the gospels. I began to pray that the enemy would not have anything in me, that he would have no claim on me, and that there would not be any open doors for him in my life. I wanted to be like Yeshua. So, in that, I gave (and continue to give) the Ruach HaKodesh the permission to put a finger on anything in my life that keeps me from wholeness and completeness. It is important to know that things in the spiritual kingdoms are all based on legal order. The adversary cannot affect us without a legal right obtained in the courts of the King of Kings. Why do you think he is noted as the *"...the accuser of our brothers and sisters—the one who accuses them before our God day and night..."* (Revelation 12:10). Where is he accusing us? In the courtroom of heaven.

Sometimes the Ruach HaKodesh speaks to me through my prayers for others. I find while praying for another person, the words that come forth will surprise me. I have to ponder them for myself. Sometimes they shed light on my own situation. This was one of those times. I had been tormented by periods of excessive bleeding and hemorrhaging during perimenopause. This particular period went on for seven weeks and I felt I identified with the woman mentioned in the above verse. Several times I felt the Lord had touched me, but I continued to have surprise "attacks" that would take me out physically.

One particular day, during an especially difficult episode, I was praying for another young woman who had psoriasis on her hands. As I was praying for her in other areas, I began to pray for her hands. The words *"Reveal to her what legal right the enemy has to torment her with this condition"* came out in my prayer for her. Those words arrested me. I began to wonder what legal right the enemy had to torment *me* with *my* bleeding. That evening my husband went to bed early. I felt led to stay up, seeking the Lord for an answer to my question. As I lay prostrate before Him, a memory came flooding back into my mind. I knew immediately that this was the root of my problem. It was so clear that I had opened a door to the enemy at that time. It connected the dots for me with not only these episodes of bleeding, but also a miscarriage I had had several years prior. Even though I thought I had repented of the sin connected with that memory, YHVH wanted me to confess it to my husband and have him pray for me to be healed because it involved him too. I woke him up tearfully confessing my hidden sin. He forgave me, repented as well, and we prayed together. I expected it to all be over right away, but that night I bled heavier than I ever had before. I had to rebuke the spirit of death all night long. However, by morning, I felt the lifting of the battle and the bleeding subside. I stopped having these episodes for over a year.

Have you ever wondered why someone gets healed only to have their symptoms return? It causes many questions to be raised. I don't believe there is a straight answer. I believe each person and each situation is so individual that it requires great discernment and wisdom to know the reason. Soul wounds can be so well hidden that the root cause of disease is also hidden. The enemy can try to take back territory that was won in a previous battle and he needs to be reminded that he no longer has a legal right to torment. There can be many reasons, but it does happen.

It happened to me. After a year of no periods, the textbooks say a woman has successfully completed her "change of life" and she is fully in menopause. Well, after 13 months of no periods I began menstruating again. The first several months seemed normal and stopped on their own. Then they stopped again. I thought it was just a fluke. But several months later I began to bleed again. We were in the same place I had dealt with the "legal cause" the last time. It was also at a time that I was grieving a loss and very confused as to why we were back in this place. I rebuked the enemy and declared that he had no legal right to torment me in this area. I prayed, asking the Lord for discernment because I didn't understand why this was happening again when it was supposedly taken care of 18 months prior.

The situation deteriorated to the point that I had to seek medical advice. I was told it would be a miracle if I didn't have uterine cancer. For a week I lay in bed wondering if this was the end of my life. I felt peaceful, with the presence of the Lord very near, but what surfaced was a memory of something that I had heard nearly 30 years before. We had a friend who was diagnosed with uterine or ovarian cancer, I can't remember which. I only remember that something inside said *"This is what will happen to you."* At the time I did not realize it was a lie from the enemy that was planted in my mind. I believed it. It was buried very deep. It reminds me of Job when he was suffering and said, *"...For the thing I dreaded has come upon me, and what I feared has happened to me."* (Job 3:24(25))

I repented for believing the lie. I listened to a message on blessings and began to bless my body, thanking my womb for housing my beautiful daughters and nourishing them. I spoke life into myself and my body. The test came back negative. Miraculously the bleeding stopped. This time I believe it was meant to expose that lie so that I could be freed from the underlying spiritual cause.

The Father is so gentle in how He exposes these areas of our lives. It's like layers of an onion. If we respond to the revelations He gives us, it brings us closer to Him. It frees us to be all we were purposed to be! *"For with You is the fountain of life and in Your light we see light."* (Psalm 36:10(9))

Another area the Father exposed to me more recently is the "Shame, Fear, Control" stronghold that most of us walk around with. Basically, it is inherent in humankind. When Adam and Eve disobeyed the command to "not eat" of the tree of the knowledge of good and evil and abandoned the relationship with their creator, what was the first thing they experienced? Shame. Then they were afraid. After that there was the blame game and trying to control the outcome. So, we all have this problem. We are basically born with the tendency to exhibit these same responses. Over time and with the experiences we have in our lives - which the enemy is proud to set up against us - we build a nice little castle where the enemy's cohorts take up residence, speaking the lies of shame, fear, and control into our minds so we create a whole host of possible negative responses. We certainly don't want anyone else to know that we have a struggle with these areas!

Heaven forbid! And so the enemy has us in his vice grip every time something goes against us. We put up walls or we get angry and take it out on others or we have a melt-down or we crawl in our shell or...whatever the response is that makes us feel secure – but it is all a lie. It only reinforces our feelings of abandonment.

I went through a teaching series by Chester and Betsy Kylstra from "Restoring the Foundations" ministry. It was so enlightening and freeing to simply recognize the stronghold and then be set free from its grip on my life. Through acknowledgment, repentance, and taking authority over the adversary and his cohorts, I felt a total shift in the way I viewed myself and others. I thought I was the only one in the world that struggled with shame! That is one of the biggest lies the enemy throws at us. *"You are the only one....."*

This is another area where the adversary doesn't want us to gain victory. He wants to keep us believing we are not worthy of the position the Father gave to us when we became His children. He certainly doesn't want us to claim the blood of Yeshua and its power to forgive, cleanse, heal, restore, and deliver! He doesn't even want us to believe there are any demons lurking around trying to bring us down and making us trip at every possible moment. If we can stay defeated, then we will never overcome him. But, if we learn to take the authority we have been given and learn the tools of the kingdom to overcome the powers of darkness, we will be a force to be reckoned with and the enemy will have to pack his bags and get out of Dodge! *"Yeshua summoned His twelve disciples and gave them authority over unclean spirits, so they could drive them out and heal every kind of disease and sickness."* (Matthew 10:1) If we are His disciples then we have been given the same authority and not only can we take authority over the adversary in our own lives, but we can assist others on their path to freedom too! How cool is that!

Questions to consider:

Are there any open doors to the enemy in my life? Is there anything in my house that could be of an occult nature? – Any books, movies, artifacts that could carry a demonic spirit? Do I or have I ever participated in Halloween or other pagan rituals and holidays? What about generational curses or consequences for the sins of our fathers? (Exodus 34:7) Do I need to cut them off and find healing and deliverance? (Freemasonry, witchcraft, other inheritances)

Am I willing to allow the Holy Spirit to expose any areas of darkness in my life so I can be set free?

Am I willing to repent of past sins and ask the Holy Spirit to show me memories and events that might have allowed the enemy a "legal right" to torment me?

What lies have I believed from the enemy? What is the truth?

Am I an "accuser of the brethren" instead of an encourager?

Do I realize the authority I have been given and do I use it?

What have I learned from this treasure?

~ Treasure #9 ~

"Be still (Let go / Cease striving / Release) and know that I am God" (Psalm 46:11 (10))

The above verse has been, what I call, one of my lifelong verses. I have had to learn each separate word of that short phrase. I came from a family and heritage of "doers". We have a great work ethic. Most of us are "Type A" overachievers who strive to be hard workers, result oriented, trustworthy, and all around good people pleasers. There is nothing intrinsically wrong with that. Every type of person and personality has strengths and weaknesses. The weakness of a "doer" is that we have trouble just "being". In our striving we have difficulty being still long enough to catch our breath. We have to always be doing something! We feel the weight of the world's problems on our shoulders and we care about everything and everyone. On top of that we would like to save everyone and fix it all. So, we often burn out and can end up sick from our "doing" and striving. We are not "at rest". As they say, *"Been there – done that."*

If we look at the first word of the above verse in the original Hebrew language, it is "rafa" (resh,pey/fey,hey – רפה) which means "to cast down, let fall, let go, relax." The word "rafa" used in the verse is very close to the Hebrew word for "heal, healer" "rafa" (resh, pey/fey, aleph רפא). YHVH knows that when we let go, release, and relax, we find healing!

When we hold on to things, we are trying to control them. We can be holding on to grudges or disappointments, hurts or fears, or expectations. Whatever we are holding onto is not in the hands of YHVH. *"Throw all your anxieties (Cast all your cares) upon Him, because He cares about you."* (I Peter 5:7)

Who is God? He says *"Let go and know that I AM God."* Yes. The great **I AM**. The Elohim of Abraham, Isaac, and Jacob. The One who was and is and is to come. When we release or let go of the things we are holding onto, we are trusting YHVH. I always ask myself, *"How much do I really trust YHVH? Am I trying to control the situation or person? Is there something I need to let go of?"* It doesn't hurt to do a self-examination, asking these important questions. As I shared at the beginning from Psalm 139 *"Examine me, God and know my heart. Test me, and know my thoughts. See if there is in me any hurtful way, and lead me along the eternal ways."* (vs. 23,24)

We have enough task masters who command us to "make bricks". YHVH invites us to come into His rest. He invites us to a Sabbath, a feast, a rest. *"Come to Me, all who are weary and burdened, and I will give you rest. Take My yoke upon you and learn from Me, for I am gentle and humble in heart, and 'you will find rest for your souls.' For My yoke is easy and My burden is light."* (Matthew 11:28-30)

I love the following quote, even though it is directed toward women (who seem to strive more than men). It can be applied to anyone. *"A woman in her glory, a woman of beauty is a woman who is not striving to become beautiful, or worthy, or enough. She knows in her quiet center where God dwells that He finds her beautiful, has deemed her worthy, and in Him, she is enough. In fact, the only thing getting in the way of our being fully captivating and enjoyed is our striving. "He will quiet you with his love." (Zephaniah 3:17) A woman of true beauty is a woman, who, in the depths of her soul is at rest, trusting God, because she has come to know Him to be worthy of her trust. She exudes a sense of calm, a sense of rest, and invites those around her to rest as well. She speaks comfort. She knows that we live in a world at war, that we have a vicious enemy, and our journey is through a broken world. But, she also knows that because of God, all is well, that all will be well. A woman of true beauty offers others the*

grace to be and the room to become." (Taken from "Captivating – Unveiling the Mystery a Woman's Soul" © 2011 by John and Stasi Eldredge, page 134. Used by permission of Thomas Nelson. www.thomasnelson.com)

Questions to consider:

What are my strengths?

What are my weaknesses?

Do I strive? Do I feel I have to perform to be accepted by YHVH?

Do I have trouble just "being"? Can I rest?

Do I take a true Sabbath rest each week? Have I ever considered the Biblical model from Genesis 2 when YHVH Himself rested on the 7th day? (before the fall of man.) Have I considered the fourth commandment concerning the Sabbath?

Is there anything I am "holding onto" – like grudges, hurts, fears, expectations?

What have I learned from this treasure?

~ Treasure #10 ~

At war with Lyme disease

"Borrelial organisms are unique in the microbial world. They possess features unusual to bacteria.....The Lyme spirochetes are fast, the fastest of all the spirochetes....Once in their new host, Lyme spirochetes continually alter their structure in order to evade host immune responses and to enhance their colonization of different parts of the body......Researchers have described their capacity in this regard as "nearly inexhaustible"... They tend to live deeper within tissues than other kinds of bacteria....ticks are not the only transmitters of Lyme disease.....Infections from larvae are, in fact, more common than old-Lyme thinking would have you believe.....Unfortunately, larval ticks are tiny, about the size of the point of a pin or the period at the end of this sentence. Impossible to see, really....They alter their genomic structure so they can enter into and live within that new host, avoiding its immune responses......They act as...portable incubators...to accomplish immune evasion feats not witnessed elsewhere in the animal kingdom....Over time, it gets harder and harder for the immune cells to find the spirochetal variants....Still, the healthier the immune system is, the faster it will ultimately figure out how it's being hustled, and the sooner you get well. Importantly, in those with very healthy immune function, during infection there will often be few or no symptoms; and the body will clear the infection fairly quickly....." (excerpts from Chapter 5 "Healing Lyme" by Stephen Harrod Buhner – Raven Press- Silver City NM ©2015 – Used by permission)

"Halleluyah! Happy is the man who fears Adonai, who delights greatly in His mitzvot. His offspring will be mighty in the land. The generation of the upright will be blessed. Wealth and riches are in his house, and his righteousness endures forever. Light shines in the darkness for the upright. Gracious, compassionate and just is he. Good comes to a man who is gracious and lends. He will order his affairs with fairness. Surely he will never be shaken. The righteous are remembered forever. <u>He is not afraid of bad news—his heart is steadfast, trusting in Adonai. His heart is secure, he will not fear—until he gazes on his foes.</u>" (Psalms 112:1-8)

"Teach us to count our days so we will become wise" (Psalms 90:12 - CJB)

Despite all of the things YHVH has taught me concerning health and healing, and my daily prayers, I found myself invaded by one of the most diabolical pathogens ever created by man (or YHVH as a judgment). (It is of course a conspiracy belief, but quite substantiated that the Lyme pathogen is a man-made biological weapon created on Plum Island off the coast of Long Island.) A true pestilence regardless of its origins.

I didn't even know I had been bitten by a tick (or other source) until I saw a sore develop on my back that continued to spread around my torso until it was almost in a circumference! It was the classic "bulls eye" Lyme or Erythema Migrans rash caused by the Borrelia Burgdorferi bacteria. There was no need to do a test. There is no other pathogen that causes this type of rash.

I believe in the above verses from Psalm 112. I knew I was in serious trouble with this invasion, but I decided that I would not "be afraid of bad news". I declared that I did not "have" Lyme disease, but was only "at war" with it. It was not going to defeat me! I was going to defeat it! With the help of YHVH, of course. Here is where all the treasures in my treasure chest were tested and used. I knew that I had to build up my immune system and find ways to attack the Lyme pathogen in every way possible. We didn't have a doctor and continued to have no health insurance. I sought YHVH diligently to know what to do. I felt that the natural antibiotic of Colloidal Silver was the first line of defense because I researched what I was dealing with and found out that the bacteria can "encyst" itself and hide with conventional antibiotics which often leads to Chronic Lyme Disease. I asked YHVH how much to take every day. I researched natural remedies and purchased some of them as I felt led. Then I knew I had to find a doctor because the Lord told me it was time to take regular antibiotics. Where would I go? Who would be the right doctor for this situation? Would he be "Lyme literate"? Would he yell at me for using natural remedies? Who? Where? I kept praying and asking YHVH to reveal this rare person to me. One day our landlord mentioned a doctor in the area he went to one time. I felt led to call his office. My two questions; *"Does he deal with Lyme disease?"* And *"Will he have a problem with me taking natural remedies"* were answered with *"Every day"* and *"No problem."* If I could have made a list of everything I would look for in a doctor, I could not have found someone who "fit the bill" as well as this doctor did. Amazing! And he was only about 10 miles away! He did confirm my self-diagnosis and prescribed a month long antibiotic regimen. I continued to take various natural remedies as recommended by the above quoted book "Healing Lyme". As I read that book, which is quite clinical, I discovered that I was dealing with a pathogen unlike any ever discovered in the natural realm! I was truly at war with the very powers of darkness whether allowed by YHVH or created by man.

Over the past year I have continued my war. For the most part I feel well and have only one slight symptom which I continue to monitor. I continue to believe it will rectify itself over time. I continue to believe I will conquer this disease with my faith and trust in YHVH and of course His help and mercy!

I realize that I am a part of a fallen world and my body is subject to the path of all men. Yeshua said that in this world we would have tribulation, but He had overcome the world. (John 16:33) I will continue to proclaim that *"All is well, All will be well."*

I am determined to live out my life to the fullness of what has been given to me. I will continue to give YHVH my mind, will, and emotions each day. I will continue to command my soul to Bless YHVH. I will continue to command my body to bow the knee to the Lordship of Yeshua and come into alignment with the will of YHVH. I will continue to bind the spiritual powers of darkness, including infirmity and cancel every assignment the enemy has against me and my family. I will continue to claim the promises of Psalm 91 and 121. I will continue to begin my day in praise and thanksgiving to the giver of life. *"I will bless the Lord at all times, His praise shall continually be in my mouth!"* (Psalm 34:1)

I saw a book one time entitled *"You Can Fear God – Or – Everything Else"*. I choose to fear Elohim. How about you?

Questions to consider:

Do I "have" a disease or am I "at war" against it?

Do I proclaim that "All is well, all will be well"?

Am I content to have YHVH direct my steps even if they lead me through the "valley of the shadow of death"?

Do I trust YHVH completely?

Do I "fear" YHVH or do I fear everything else?

What have I learned from this treasure?

~ Conclusion ~

If.....Then...

"Loved ones, I pray that all may go well with you and that you may be in good health, just as it is well with your soul. For I was overjoyed when some brethren came and testified of the truth in you—how you are walking in truth. I have no greater joy than this—to hear that my children are walking in the truth." (3 John 1:2-4)

"If you listen closely to what Adonai your God says, observing and obeying all his mitzvoth* (commandments) which I am giving you today, ...all the following blessings will be yours in abundance - if you do what Adonai your God says;..........But if you refuse to pay attention to what Adonai your God says, and do not observe and obey all his mitzvoth and regulations which I am giving you today, then all the following curses will be yours in abundance........." (Deuteronomy 28 - CJB)

"You are to serve Adonai your God, and He will bless your food and your water. Moreover I will take sickness away from your midst. None will miscarry nor be barren in your land, and I will fill up the number of your days." (Exodus 23:25-26)

I believe YHVH desires for us to be well, in every area of our lives. His plan is for us to believe that what He says is true and obey it so that He can bless us! The above verse in 3 John indicates and confirms that our physical health is connected to our spiritual health – the health of our "soul". In the Deuteronomy passages we see that it also depends on our obedience to His commandments. This is not "name it, claim it" prosperity teaching, nor is it "have to" or "under the law" doctrine! This is a Want To – Get To follow YHVH's instructions (Torah) because I love Him with my whole heart, soul, mind, and strength! This is living Biblically! This is recognizing that YHVH says *"If you will…. Then I will….."* We can't claim the "then" if we don't do the "if"! We can't presume upon His graces.

In recent years I have rediscovered the *treasures* in YHVH's word and the Hebrew roots of my faith. Along that journey I have come to understand that my Christian heritage has been deprived of some of the most profound blessings that YHVH desires us to have. When we lost the Biblical Sabbath, and the Feasts of YHVH we lost some amazing blessings that come with their observance (and a whole lot of no-guilt rest!). For example, on the Sabbath, we bring the day "in" Friday at sundown with a family feast. The wife blesses the husband. The husband blesses the wife and then the children are all individually or corporately blessed. If our households were raised with such blessings spoken out over us week after week as well as the weekly Torah readings, I believe we would not have the breakdown in family that we see today. The feasts are also times of great blessings. Following the Torah (instructions) of YHVH from Genesis 1 to Revelation 22 is vital to receiving these blessings. We cannot pick and choose which commandments we want to follow. Everything is there for a reason. If we don't understand it – we need to go to the author and ask.

There are unending *treasures* to be discovered in the living Word of Elohim. May I invite you to seek His face, read His word, find out for yourself what may be lacking in your understanding and dig for more? *"Don't be conceited about your own wisdom; but fear Adonai and turn from evil. This will bring health to your body and give strength to your bones."* (Proverbs 3:7,8) *"… for they are life to those who find them and health to their whole being."* (Proverbs 4:22) *"Those who love your Torah have great shalom, nothing makes them stumble."* (Psalm 119:165 and so many more wonderful verses in that Psalm!) *"Far more blessed are those*

52

who hear the word of God and obey it!" (Yeshua in Luke 11:28) and finally *"Because you are listening to these rulings, keeping and obeying them, Adonai your God will keep with you the covenant and mercy that He swore to your ancestors. He will love you, bless you, and increase your numbers; He will also bless the fruit of your body, and the fruit of your ground.......there will not be a sterile male or female among you and the same with your livestock. Adonai will remove all illness from you....."* (Deuteronomy 7:11-15)

For I know the plans that I have in mind for you," declares Adonai, *"plans for shalom and not calamity—to give you a future and a hope. "Then you will call on Me, and come and pray to Me, and I will listen to you. You will seek Me and find Me, when you will search for Me with all your heart.* (Jeremiah 29:11-13)

****

But.... what *"IF"* you have done all you can and you are not healed? *"THEN"*, we must **JUST STAND** as so aptly put in this song.

Weeping only lasts a night. How long will this night be?
In the shadow of your burdens, it's hard for you to see.
Though the trials you may face
    may bring you to your knees.
There's no better place for you to be.
Then at the end of your ability.

Chorus:
When you've done all you can to Stand - Stand on Him
Though all the world around is sinking sand.
When it seems that you just can't go on,
In your weakness He'll be strong.
When you feel like you've done everything you can,
Just Stand

If it seems there's one more mountain,
One more war to fight.
One more time you feel forsaken.
There's no hope in sight.
Remember where He's brought you from,
And what He's brought you through.
There's nothing that's too hard for God to do.
For through it all He's always seen you through.
(Chorus)

Stand upon His promises.
Stand upon His word.
Every step He takes with you.
Every prayer He's heard. (Chorus)

When you feel like you've done everything you can.
When you feel that you have finally reached the end.
When you feel like you've done everything you can.
Just stand - Just stand - You just stand.

I pleaded with the Lord three times about this, that it might leave me. But He said to me, "My grace is sufficient for you, for power is made perfect in weakness." Therefore I will boast all the more gladly in my weaknesses, so that the power of Messiah may dwell in me. For Messiah's sake, then, I delight in weaknesses, in insults, in distresses, in persecutions, in calamities. For when I am weak, then I am strong. (2 Corinthians 12:8-10)

Questions to consider:

What do I need to change in my life to become healthier?

Am I willing to re-examine all the "commandments" and see what wisdom is in its teaching?

Do I have any areas where I am in disobedience to YHVH's commandments or personal commands?

Am I willing to re-examine widely accepted beliefs to see if I am truly "walking in truth"?

What if I never get the healing and answers I am looking for? Will I "stand" on His promises and trust YHVH? Will I accept that in my weakness He is strong?

What are the personal "treasures" YHVH has already taught me?

What have I learned from this whole teaching on Treasures Toward Wholeness?

Natural Remedy "tools" I always have on hand*

Arnica gel or cream – bruises, injury, sprains (never on open wound- but you can buy homeopathic subcutaneous pills)

Astragalus – (1000 mg) Supplement to have on hand during Tick season. Boosts immune system and fights against Lyme.

Bentonite Clay – a natural clay from special volcanic ash that draws poisons out of your system. You can purchase food grade for an internal cleanse or use it on insect bites and poison ivy as a poultice. Good for IBS/digestive problems.

Chaparral Red Clover Salve – for pre-cancer spots. Kills the bad cells. (Taylormadearomatherapy.com)

Colloidal Silver – natural antibiotic – liquid – safe for all ages and infections (including MRSA!) (Research Quality and type!!)

Diatomaceous Earth – a natural powder from places where the ocean used to be. The "diatoms" scrub your internal digestive system and liver. It can even remove heavy metals, parasites, and pesticides. Also good for skin, bones, nails and any part of your body that needs/utilizes silica. Good for household bug infestations too!

Echinacea Tea – boosts the immune system

Golden Seal Myrrh salve – any skin abrasions, infections, or burns. (Taylormadearomatherapy.com/HerbalSalves/Goldenseal_Myrrh_Salve.html)

Pau d'arco – (I buy bulk shredded bark) - Antiviral tea for flu/cold symptoms. Boil about ¼ cup for 5 minutes in 4 cups water. Drink at least 4 cups first day you feel any symptoms of "coming down with something". May drink for 2-3 days. Not effective if already sick or for bacterial infections. "Nip it in the bud" as Barney Fife would say.

Rescue Remedy (Dr. Bach's) – stress, anxiety, fear, travel – works great on animals too.

* Concerning the Natural Remedies listed: These statements have not been evaluated by the Food and Drug Administration.